MEDITATION NOT MEDICINE

Survive and Thrive
in Our Stress-Filled World

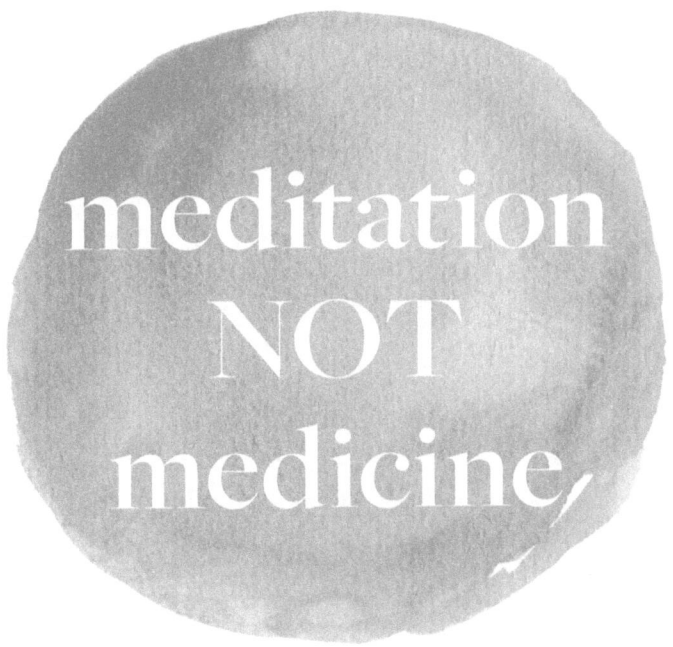

meditation NOT medicine

Adam J. Weber

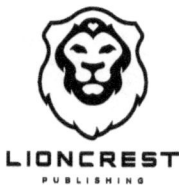

COPYRIGHT © 2021 ADAM J. WEBER

All rights reserved.

MEDITATION NOT MEDICINE

Survive and Thrive in Our Stress-Filled World

ISBN 978-1-5445-1836-7 *Hardcover*
      978-1-5445-1835-0 *Paperback*
      978-1-5445-1834-3 *Ebook*

I would like to dedicate this book to you. I am grateful for your time and your trust in me. Your time is a precious commodity, and I promise not to waste it.

Contents

Running on Empty 9
The Take-a-Pill Approach 15
The Meditation Approach 19
What to Expect 23
Change and Action 25
Start with an Intention 27
The Epidemic of Stress 31
Stress, Mental Health, and Physical Health 37
Stress, Chronic Illness, and Pain 41
When the World Falls Apart 43
The Do-Nothing Mindset 47
Responding, Not Reacting 51
What Is Meditation? 55
What Can Meditation Do for You? 57
A Quiet Mind 59
Better Rest and Sleep 61
Meditation, Anxiety, and Depression 63

Meditation and Physical Health.................................... 67
High Blood Pressure 69
Your Immune System 71
Meditation, Chronic Illness, and Pain 73
Meditation, Relationships, and Quality of Life 75
Meditation and Crisis 77
How to Get the Most from Your Meditation Practice.. 79
Consistently Meditating... 81
When Should You Meditate? 85
How Long and How Often Should You Meditate?....... 87
Where to Meditate... 91
The Meditation Practice 93
Creating a Habit 97
The Monkey Mind...101
When You Hit a Wall..103
Getting Support..105
Almost Done 107
Acknowledgments... 111
About the Author.. 113

Running on Empty

My days in the corporate world usually started at 3:00 a.m., when it was still dark outside but I was wide awake.

Day after day, weekends too, I was overwhelmed. It was like putting my foot on the gas pedal and being unable to find the brake to slow down or stop.

My body would ache to go back to sleep for just fifteen more minutes, but I would wake up, and my adrenaline would be pumping. The anticipation of a full day, being pulled in twenty different directions, woke me up.

I had a wife and worked in commercial real estate for one of the world's real estate giants. The corporate world in New York City is well known for serving up stress on a silver platter. I made great money, but I let the work own me.

The stress was eating me alive, and I was hurting bad.

I became easily agitated, frustrated, and moody. At times I not only felt like I was losing control; at times, I *did* lose control. I had difficulty relaxing. I felt lonely, worthless, and depressed. I avoided others like they were the plague, including those closest to me.

My health was a mess. I had knee surgery and then back surgery for two herniated discs. But what was supposed to be a routine double discectomy turned into much more.

My doctor, a neurologist, asked me to come to his office for a follow-up visit. At the appointment, he pulled up my MRI and X-rays.

He pointed out numerous spots to me on the film. They were lesions on my spine, and they were from multiple sclerosis.

Multiple sclerosis is an incurable and debilitating disease. Multiple sclerosis is a life sentence.

Stress exacerbates the symptoms of multiple sclerosis, and at times my stress became unmanageable. At times I was unable to eat or walk without falling. Everyday tasks became hard to do. It became tough to work in my hard-charging job, and my relationships suffered, both personally and professionally.

You might be in the same position as I was: working hard, raising your family, and doing twenty other things at any given time. You might, as I was, be facing a chronic illness made even worse by stress. You might feel anxious or depressed because of your stress. You might be struggling to meet the overwhelming demands of the present world. I've been there.

You wake up every day, and the stress hits the fan. You go home after work, and the stress hits the fan. Weekends and holidays come, and the stress hits the fan. But how do you cope?

My diagnosis forced me to figure it out. I had no choice. After speaking with my doctors and conducting exhaustive research, I finally had the proverbial aha moment.

My breakthrough: meditation! With meditation, I was

able to reduce my stress and calm my mind, even in the midst of incredibly challenging circumstances. I was able to see improvements in my pain and symptoms. You can too.

It is no secret that stress is one of the most common conditions in the world. Millions of people are suffering from stress this very minute, but the good news is that the suffering can end.

It doesn't matter who you are or where you live. Stress doesn't care about your age or your net worth. Nothing is worse than walking through your own big, dark, and violent stress tsunami. Fortunately, you don't have to be thrown around by the tsunami anymore. Stress can be managed, lessened, and tamed through meditation. When the stress lightens, everything else gets easier.

A daily meditation practice can address your stress, reduce your anxiety, improve some of your physical ailments and pain, and give you a higher quality of life. You can enjoy a better, calmer life where you feel more in control and more able to cope.

When I started meditating many years ago, I was nervous. Meditation was new to me, and I had no idea what I should expect. I wondered if meditation was supposed to be like an off switch for my stress. I had no clear expectations, and it seemed there were no guarantees with anything.

I read books about meditation and ran into so much flowery woo-woo fluff. I wish that someone had just given me simple, actionable information. I ended up writing the book I wish I had then.

The reality was different than expected. Within days of starting to meditate, I felt the stress start to melt away. The benefits began compounding, and soon I no longer felt on edge. As of the writing of this book, I have practiced meditation for more than ten years. It has helped me in many ways, but most importantly in reducing my own internal stress and anxiety. It has given me a drug-free tool that I can use as often as needed, anytime and anywhere.

There are six recognized types of meditation, including the three I have personally utilized: mindfulness meditation, focused meditation, and transcendental meditation. Most are needlessly difficult for the beginner. Given how incredibly effective meditation is to control stress, and how common the epidemic of stress has become, it is time for that to change. I wrote this book to be of service, to offer a framework that truly makes it easy for anyone to meditate.

You may not be as stressed as I was or dealing with the same physical symptoms from the stress, but you deserve an answer. You deserve a solution that won't cause you more stress or any of the troubling side effects of medication.

The Take-a-Pill Approach

My father was an old-school doctor who would hand me a pill every time I burped, coughed, or passed gas.

He had been taught to give patients a pill for everything, and then everything would be just fine. That is an old and tired approach to practicing medicine and helping people.

When you have a medical problem, do you automatically look for the quick fix with a pill? My research indicates that with our increasingly busy lifestyles, we tend to opt for the quick fix, but it has costs.

It has been reported that approximately 30 percent of us have used two or more prescription drugs in the past thirty days, and more than 10 percent of us have used five or more. Many of us may even be using over-the-counter drugs alongside these. But do we know what this medication is doing to our health?

Not only is the take-a-pill approach not a consistent, reliable way to reduce your stress, but it can also be toxic. Even though most pills are supposed to be safe, nearly all come with side effects and some come with real problems. Complications from most medications are rare, but they happen, and they can be serious. Medications may have unpredictable effects when taken. Taking pills necessarily comes with risk.

I appreciate the role that medical professionals play in helping people overcome their illnesses, but let me be clear: I do not personally agree with some of their approaches or solutions. And unfortunately, the take-a-pill approach is the common approach.

On the other hand, it is common knowledge that a lifestyle change can help significantly with stress without the side effects—a lifestyle change that includes meditation practice, not more medicine.

The potential of a meditation practice should not

be underestimated. Science has proven it effective. Studies conducted at the University of Wisconsin and elsewhere have shown that meditation has physiological effects on the brain. Researchers found that when meditation is practiced regularly and consistently, the part of the brain that regulates stress and anxiety shrinks. Numerous health benefits come with developing a regular meditation practice, some of which can be felt quickly after people start meditating.

Doctors, mental health experts, counselors, and other professionals are important in helping you overcome the personal challenges you face. However, they are not enough, and some of their solutions come with inherent risk. Meditation is nontoxic and cheap, and it has only positive effects.

My positions are clear. Anyone can take a pill if they have a doctor who will prescribe one, but even better, anyone can practice meditation. No prescription is required. Meditation is simple and inexpensive, and it doesn't require any special equipment.

And you can practice meditation wherever you are. It doesn't matter whether you are out for a walk, riding the bus, waiting at the doctor's office, or even in the middle of a difficult business meeting.

Why not meditate?

The Meditation Approach

Meditation is a natural, drug-free, cost-effective solution to address your stress. It requires just minutes per day.

Studies have shown that meditation induces your relaxation response. According to an article published in *Forbes* magazine in 2015, research illustrates that meditation has an amazing variety of neurological benefits, from positive changes in gray-matter volume to reduced activity in the "me" centers of the brain to enhanced connectivity among brain regions. There is evidence that meditation helps relieve our levels of anxiety and depression. It can improve attention, concentration, and overall psychological well-being.

Meditation decreases anxiety and depression. It increases resiliency. Many practitioners report a deep sense of inner peace, much less stress, and a greater sense of well-being.

With less stress, you will improve your relationships and embrace a better quality of life. Without the weight of stress, you are likely to see improvements in your health.

Meditation can improve the quality of your life. It can give you a sense of calm, peace, and balance that can benefit both your emotional well-being and your overall health.

For some, the benefits of meditation happen right away. For others, it takes more time.

According to Mindworks, the issue of how long it takes for our practice to "work" becomes irrelevant when we realize that meditation is a lifelong commitment. The early stages of a meditation practice can be a tad frustrating. The mind flutters and wanders about, the slightest disturbance throws us off, and unwelcome thoughts pester us annoyingly. But with time, we stop struggling with these issues and start looking forward to our daily meditation.

However, just because you meditate, it doesn't mean you will never be stressed again. Sadly, life doesn't work this way.

What to Expect

This book will give you the step-by-step approach to relaxing your mind and beating your stress through the meditation technique that I have developed, called Easy to Meditate.

People find it hard to meditate for all sorts of reasons. Easy to Meditate is different than other techniques, and it really *is* easy. With Easy to Meditate, there are no difficult postures to sit in. There are no difficult or unnatural mantras to remember and chant. And most importantly, there are no hard-set rules. Easy to Meditate is a practice that can be customized and adjusted to fit your needs and what you are comfortable doing.

This book is for those who are willing to take action and devote just minutes a day to self-care and dealing with stress.

In this book, you will find a process that you can implement into your life easily and that will take your stress-reduction efforts to the next level.

I've made the book intentionally short, practical, and results-oriented. To get the most out of it, you have to take consistent action. If you do, your ability to work with your stress will get better, which will improve your life.

Change and Action

Change isn't easy. To see results, you're required to get out of your comfort zone and embrace the unknown. You must take consistent, massive action on what you've learned, even if it seems hard to find the time. Meditation takes minutes per day, but without those minutes, you won't see results.

This is your new beginning. I am here to meet you where you are. I am privileged to be your guide and to walk with you step-by-step. However, meditation won't work if you don't take action.

Go to www.meditationnotmedicine.com and join the community there, which can provide support for you on your journey.

Start with an Intention

As you read this book and implement its strategies, I ask that you begin with the end in mind.

Your first step is to clearly understand your current pain, your current stress, and the source or sources of your stress.

To understand your stress better, you must understand that there are different stress levels and that these levels vary in the form they take. The point at which stress becomes a problem is different for everyone. When the negative emotions and feelings of stress inhibit your ability to live a happy and healthy life, stress is having a significant negative effect on you. According to the Mental Health Foundation (2009), you need to recognize the physical warnings such as tense muscles, overtiredness, headaches, or migraines that may be a result of stress. If any of the symptoms of stress—emotional, behavioral, physical, or mental—become too much for an individual to handle and cope with in everyday life, stress has become a problem.

When you have recognized that you're suffering because of stress, you then need to identify the underlying causes and triggers. Understanding what causes you to become stressed allows you to identify ways to manage it, either by avoiding those triggers or reducing the impact of those stressful events. It is also important to realize that when you are already stressed, the number of triggers and causes also increases. Therefore, it is crucial to identify the underlying cause of your stress, not just the other factors that increase stress or are a result of an already stressful lifestyle.

Next, you need to set a goal. Without a goal, you will lack focus and direction. A goal will provide a benchmark for determining whether you are succeeding. Take a moment and think about why you want to set a meditation goal. How will achieving your meditation goal serve you and those around you?

Now, let us set that goal.

First, consider what goal you want to achieve, be specific about it, and then commit to achieving it. Why do you want this goal? Be clear and decide the price you are willing to pay to achieve it.

You must write down your goal. Put pen to paper and write it down. Put this note in a prominent place. Put it in multiple places.

Think about your goal and act on it every day.

The Epidemic of Stress

We live in a time of unprecedented, constant change—coronavirus, global warming, evolving technology, death and divorce, business failings and successes—all leading to major stress. Yet many are at a loss as to how to deal with their stress in a healthy way. We are all constantly on the brink of exhaustion, distraction, procrastination, depression, and more. Stress is hurting us.

You may be stressed because you have had a change in your life, such as a new baby, a new job, or a financial struggle.

You may have had a trauma-filled childhood, or you may have an abusive spouse. You may be dealing with daily stressors such as traffic, bills, family, work, or an illness. We all face stress every day, day in, day out.

We live in a fast-paced world that involves us continuously looking at a screen, scrambling to get somewhere, or racing for the next appointment. From our long hours working to our home lives, it is no wonder that we are stressed out.

According to the Mental Health Foundation, stress can be defined as the degree to which you feel overwhelmed or unable to cope as a result of pressures that are unmanageable.

My definition is a bit more comprehensive and based on my research. Stress is a feeling of emotional or physical tension. It can come from an event or thought that makes you feel frustrated, angry, or nervous. Stress is your body's reaction to a challenge or demand. In short bursts, stress can be positive, such as when it helps you avoid danger or meet a deadline.

However, over a longer time frame, stress hurts our relationships, our physical and mental health, and our quality of life. It costs us financially, with lost opportunities and spiraling healthcare costs. It hurts us physically. It hurts our work and our society.

According to The American Institute of Stress, work-related stress causes 120,000 deaths and results in $190 billion in healthcare costs yearly.

Stress can be caused by numerous factors, but work often isn't the main culprit.

Long hours, work overload, productivity targets, tight deadlines, and challenging coworkers and supervisors are all well-known contributors to stress at work. It may be tempting for employers to focus on managing these areas. But personal circumstances can often be the biggest cause of stress. The breakdown of relationships, challenging dependents, falling behind in financial obligations, and poor health can all be major causes of stress and affect employees in the workplace and throughout their lives.

Our stress and anxiety are in oversupply, and we are struggling to cope. They are out of control. Yet the old model of care for treating those living with stress is broken. Mainstream medicine leaves many with little hope and even fewer answers.

Stress doesn't have to be like a backpack of bricks we haul around every day. We can learn to relax and put down the weight. We can learn to handle stress in a constructive rather than a destructive way.

Meditation affects the body in exactly the opposite ways that stress does. According to numerous studies, meditation triggers the body's relaxation response. It restores the body to a calm state, helping the body repair itself and preventing new damage from the physical effects of stress.

Can you imagine finally waking up each day without your stress grabbing and shaking you like a rag doll?

You might be surprised at how stress impacts your life. Here are some of the ways stress affects you:

1. Stress can impact your physical health. According to the American Heart Association, stress can contribute to ulcers, irritable bowel syndrome, and high blood pressure.
2. Stress can negatively impactyour mental health because it changes your brain circuitry for the worse.
3. Relationships can suffer when you feel a lot of

stress in your life. Your stress response can badly impact how you treat others.

4. How well do you do at work when you are stressed out? If your stress and anxiety keep you up at night, you won't be effective at your job.
5. All the areas that stress impacts relate to the quality of life. When you have a lot of stress and there is a lot of negativity because of it, it can ruin your life.
6. The greater the stress, the greater the likelihood that you will make bad decisions. Knee-jerk reactions can cause you to make risky or premature decisions. You will drop long-range goals for immediate survival needs, and every day you will wonder why you keep falling behind instead of getting ahead.
7. Stress locks you into fight, flight, or freeze reactions. Your emotional set point switches to a negative setting, predisposing you to anxiety, anger, aggression, paranoia, and depression.
8. Chronic stress impairs your immune system, and it wreaks havoc on your cardiovascular system. It kills brain cells and, if left unchecked, can eventually kill you. If you add up all the deaths from stress-related illnesses, you have our number-one killer.

We often think our problems produce the stress we experience, but it is actually the reverse. Stress causes most of our troubles, from money, family, and work problems to physical and mental health issues.

If you want a healthy, happy, and successful life, controlling stress belongs at the top of your to-do list.

Eighty-three percent of us are doing nothing about our stress. Why? Stress is life-threatening. It is not something that maybe someday you should do something about. You need to address it today.

Stress, Mental Health, and Physical Health

Do you ever have moments of overwhelm? Do you ever let that overwhelm become a full-blown stress storm?

According to The American Institute of Stress, stress and depression lead to $51 billion in lost work costs due to absenteeism and $26 billion in treatment costs.

The pandemic at the time of this writing is only making anxiety and depression worse. According to an article in *Forbes*, recently completed studies, including one at Purdue University, show that the pandemic and the resulting quarantine have affected the mental health of workers at every echelon of the career ladder. A Gallup study found that due to stresses related to the pandemic, employees are 20 percent less likely to say they are well prepared to do their jobs now than prior to the pandemic.

Morneau Shepell surveyed five thousand employees between May 29 and June 9, 2020. The findings are published in the latest Mental Health Index, outlining the state of mental health among American workers. It demonstrates heightened concern about returning to pre-pandemic life among the population. The June report marked the third consecutive month with a negative mental health score. The findings show that even with parts of the country reopening, feelings of isolation remain the top threat to American employees' mental health.

Stress affects not only mental health but also physical health. If stress is a part of your everyday life, you should be concerned about your health and wellbeing. Stress is an indirect cause for more deaths per year than all the terrorist attacks and wars on this planet.

According to the journal *Stress and Physical Health* in

2017, the ten leading causes of death in the United States were, in rank order, diseases of heart; malignant neoplasms; accidents (unintentional injuries); chronic lower respiratory diseases; cerebrovascular diseases; Alzheimer's disease; diabetes mellitus; influenza and pneumonia; nephritis, nephrotic syndrome, and nephrosis; and intentional self-harm (suicide). The ten leading causes accounted for 74 percent of all deaths occurring in the United States. Notice how many of those causes of death are directly or indirectly caused by stress.

Meditation fights stress and helps restore physical and mental health. Studies have shown that meditation induces your relaxation response, which reduces your blood pressure and in turn affects levels of stress.

Stress, Chronic Illness, and Pain

Do you suffer from chronic pain or illness? Stress can be making it worse.

Research from Loma Linda University has shown that individuals who are under constant stress experience negative brain effects, including a decrease of brain function, a lowered IQ, and increased pain due to altered brain chemicals. More pain, more stress. More stress, more pain.

According to research, stress-related psychiatric disorders, which include depression and post-traumatic stress disorder (PTSD), are highly widespread, disabling illnesses with limited treatment options and poorly understood pathophysiology. Adding stress to them makes them worse.

Chronic pain affects 20–30 percent of adults, and stress makes it worse. Although numerous treatment options are available, almost half of pain-suffering individuals don't achieve adequate pain management.

Pain and stress are two distinguished yet overlapping processes that make each other worse.

When the World Falls Apart

I am finishing the writing of this book in the first half of 2020, when most of us are shaken because our lives have been changed and will never be the same again.

The COVID-19 crisis has had an impact on every corner of our lives—socializing, shopping, schooling, working, and traveling, to name a few. It has caused massive stress around the world.

As is true of any crisis, this virus will move us in one of two directions: forward or backward.

Fear took over when the coronavirus broke out. The lockdowns turned off sectors of the economy and of our lives. Unemployment rates skyrocketed, with many jobs lost permanently. After the death of George Floyd, our televisions were flooded with images of protests and civil and political unrest. This has just added to the daily stress we were already under.

The landscape as we knew it has changed for good. It is natural and logical to have some stress when the world falls apart. If you are going through another crisis at this moment, it is natural and logical to have stress now.

The uncertainty and the unknown often cause us to draw conclusions that are both negative and stressful. However, negative thoughts and emotions are dangerous. They can cause us to go backward because they can cause us to make bad decisions. As humans, we worry and stress about things that have not happened yet, but most of the time, the worst-case scenario doesn't happen, and then we breathe a massive sigh of relief. Afterward, we realize all the worry, fear, anxiety, and stress was for nothing.

However, sometimes the worst does happen.

Personally, battling a progressive form of multiple sclerosis and living a hard-charged life in the corporate world and as a business owner can trigger a tsunami of stress, and as a result, I needed an alternative to just taking another pill. That approach doesn't work.

Current events, such as the COVID-19 pandemic and political protests, have left people feeling many intense emotions—such as fear, anxiety, and anger—and generally stressed overall. Over time, that unrelenting stress has left many feeling emotionally tired and numb.

History has a habit of repeating itself, which means that in the future, we are going to face many more crises. Not all of them will be global. Some will be some local, and some will be personal.

These crises may be personal, be professional, or belong to someone we love and care about. I have found that my sound, daily meditation practice sets me up to deal with almost anything.

Meditation has taught me that I have an internal shut-off switch, and taking a seat and meditating can help me quickly and effectively deal with stress when it rears its ugly head.

Within every crisis lies an opportunity for us to grow stronger, wiser, and more resilient.

Meditation has done that for me, and it can do that for you.

The Do-Nothing Mindset

In a recent conversation, a client named Gina said she was frustrated because her stress was overwhelming her. Gina is a C-Suite executive in the New York City area.

I asked her how often she had been meditating. The phone line went silent, and then Gina, in an embarrassed tone, told me she had been able to meditate only once in the past week. She then proceeded to tell me that she was so busy at work and that she did not have any time. Frustrated, Gina told me that she has three kids, a house that requires constant cleaning, and a husband who is also a C-Suite executive and works all the time. She told me that she was too busy to meditate. Her response is, unfortunately, common.

I've often wondered why so many people complain about their stress but do not do anything about it. Those who do nothing are missing the chance to live a better-quality life and are instead stuck in an endless loop of stress. But they do nothing.

The do-nothing mindset comes from years of being programmed that we should either live with the stress or visit a doctor for a pill.

For too many, the take-a-pill approach is the easy one, but it is a bad one. Pills can provide some people with temporary results, and for others, no results at all. Another problem with the pill approach is that it can be toxic.

Stress is headed your way, whether you like it or not. It is a part of life, and no one is immune from it. Some stress is predictable, and some stress is not. Some stress can be overwhelming. When you are stressed, you may experience many different feelings, including anxiety, fear, anger, sadness, or frustration. These feelings can sometimes feed on one another and produce physical symptoms, making you feel even worse. For some people, stressful life events can contribute to symptoms of depression.

However, as humans, we are smart enough to see stress coming, and we can change our response.

Responding, Not Reacting

You have probably heard the saying "It's not what happens that matters but how you respond to what happens that matters."

The difference between those who suffer because of their stress and those who do not is how they respond to their stress. Notice that I said *respond*, not *react*.

Often when we are in the middle of a stressful situation, we don't respond appropriately, and things spiral downward from there. In other words, we do nothing or we do the wrong thing, and that only sets us back and causes a compound effect of the stress. The fallout can be negative.

When you come face-to-face with your stress, let that be your cue to respond the correct way.

The following is a transformational formula that plays an impactful role in many lives every day:

$$E + R = O$$
Event + Response = Outcome

- EVENTS are what happen to us.
- RESPONSES are how we respond to these events.
- OUTCOMES are the result of our responses to those events.

When people don't like the outcome they are experiencing, many choose to blame the event for their lack of results or the outcome. We have grown used to and comfortable with reacting, not responding, to our stress.

It is true that factors exist and that they impact you. However, if those factors were the deciding ones in whether someone succeeded, nobody would ever succeed. For every reason success isn't possible, hundreds of people have faced the same circumstances and succeeded.

So, to connect this to stress, when you feel stress, you must respond and not react by getting angry or upset.

I learned this formula from Jack Canfield as I read his classic *The Success Principles*. Everything you do is a result of your choices. Your outcome is up to you. You get to choose your response, and you must respond the right way to get the outcome you want.

The right way to address your stress is to stop, breathe, and take a seat to meditate. No rage, no food or alcohol binges. Just take a seat and meditate.

When you allow stress to take control of your mind, your body, and your life, you allow a harmful chain reaction. You react, and your body goes into stress mode. Your heart pumps your stress hormones throughout your system. You want to stop those hormones from racing through your body and causing damage. Stress hormones and their consequences cause damage. Stress is one of the leading causes of death.

As the rest of the world stays full of stress and anxiety, you can do something about it. You MUST anticipate that stress is going to come your way, whether you like it or not. If you don't anticipate that stress will come, you will feel out of control.

Unfortunately, humans are naturally programmed to react and not respond. When we react to stress, we end up making irrational or emotional decisions. Not good.

Do not allow yourself to stop and freeze. If you do, your stress and anxiety will continue to be a crisis—your crisis.

You will feel calmer when you respond properly instead of reacting. Get in the habit of responding to your stress instead of reacting to it.

Choose to respond. How can you think about what you need to do to move forward?

We live in a fast-paced and hyperconnected world—a world filled with lots of stressors. You will never fully eliminate or be 100 percent immune from your stress, but when you respond appropriately, you win.

What Is Meditation?

So what is meditation?

Meditation is defined as a practice where you use a technique, such as focusing your mind on an object, thought, or activity, to achieve a mentally clear and emotionally calm feeling inside, which some people refer to as a *state*. When you focus, you still remain in the present but focus wholly on one thing, typically sensory stimuli like sounds, visual items, tactile sensations, tastes, smells, and even your own breathing.

Meditation may be used with the aim of reducing stress, anxiety, depression, and even pain.

Meditation doesn't require any special equipment or clothes. It doesn't require you to go on any pricey retreat. If you commit 100 percent to meditating daily, you will see the results.

The history of meditation is long and rich. Meditation used to be practiced only by monks and other religious people. As its benefits have become more well known, it has grown in popularity. Today meditation is practiced by anyone who wants to address their stress and be more productive, happier, and healthier. Meditation has been proven scientifically and has become a part of the daily lives of everyday people. Doctors recommend meditation to their patients, and wellness programs have incorporated it for the same reason: its benefits.

What Can Meditation Do for You?

The first thing you might feel after meditating is just how relaxed you are. Get ready to feel better each time you meditate. As you teach your mind to relax and let go of the things that bother you, you will be able to find peace, and this, in turn, will make your life much better.

We live in a crazy world that can make it hard to focus. We also tend to live in the past, reliving our mistakes and poor choices instead of focusing on the present.

Lucky for us, meditation can help. Meditation helps us focus on the present, on what we are doing right now, not on what we were doing or will do.

A regular meditation practice changes your brain in ways that can help you control emotions, enhance concentration, decrease stress, and even become more connected to those around you. When you are more relaxed, your mind is clearer and your body is calmer. This will lead to better long-term health, wellness, and happiness.

The benefits are available to anyone who makes time to practice meditation every day.

My research has revealed that there are more than one hundred benefits to a regular meditation practice. Scientists have investigated some of the more tangible results of meditation, and the studies have revealed that meditating for even short periods of time can have positive impacts.

The biggest benefit of Easy to Meditate is that it will help you reduce the stress that can wear you out both mentally and physically. You will have more energy.

A Quiet Mind

The most valuable piece of real estate we each own is the space between our ears. Meditation increases the ability to concentrate and focus. It can encourage creativity, promote problem-solving skills, and decrease stress.

Mental clutter is the junk that takes up space in our heads and continues to live there rent-free. Meditation helps you get rid of your mental clutter. Stop being a mental hoarder, and let it go. You will feel freer. Research has shown that meditation can also help you increase your self-control for the future.

A quiet mind allows you to tap into your intuition, creativity, and energy and develop a newfound enthusiasm for life. A meditation practice empties your mind of the stories you attach to events in your life and enables you to sit with your feelings as they arise.

Better Rest and Sleep

Meditation can help you fall asleep more easily and sleep more soundly.

Harvard Health reports that meditation can help fight insomnia. Many meditators, myself included, experience better sleep.

Some people find that meditation before bed can be particularly helpful, but studies have shown that a meditation practice at any point during the day benefits our sleeping habits.

Meditation helps you to feel mentally refreshed and free from fatigue and to sleep better.

Meditation, Anxiety, and Depression

No one in life escapes event-related stress, such as the death of a loved one, the loss of a job, divorce, or even a global crisis like COVID-19.

Earlier in this book, I told you that while I was working in commercial real estate for one of the world's real estate giants, the stress was served up on a silver platter.

I was not alone. And today, if you feel this way, you are not alone.

A loss of any type is a major risk factor for depression. Grieving is considered a normal, healthy response to loss, but if it goes on for too long, it can trigger depression. A serious illness like cancer or having several autoimmune diseases is considered a chronic stressor.

Everyone has different stress triggers, and work stress tops the list, according to surveys. Forty percent of U.S. workers admit to experiencing office stress, and one-quarter say work is the biggest source of stress in their lives.

Chronic stress, in particular, leads to elevated hormones such as cortisol, the "stress hormone," and reduced serotonin and other neurotransmitters in the brain, including dopamine, which has been linked to depression.

Stress can lead to major depression in some people, and chronic stress can lead to overactivity of the body's stress-response mechanism.

Although depression is common in adults and affects about 20 percent of adults age sixty-five and older, it isn't a normal part of growing older, and it should never be taken lightly. Depression affects people's daily lives by causing them suffering and social isolation and affecting their memory. Some doctors have found that depression can be alleviated with a daily meditation practice.

A study conducted in Belgian schools found that students who practiced meditation exhibited fewer instances of depression and its related symptoms.

Studies have also shown that meditation can be helpful for retraining your brain. It has a positive effect on the emotional brain circuits.

Meditation protects the hippocampus, or the part of the brain involved in memory. People who suffer from recurrent depression tend to have a smaller hippocampus. One study discovered that people who meditated for thirty minutes a day for eight weeks increased the volume of gray matter in their hippocampus. This may explain why the Belgian schools saw less depression in those who meditated.

Meditation can also help with apprehension, anxiety, and panic. A research study published in the *American Journal of Psychiatry* showed that twenty-two patients previously diagnosed with heightened panic disorder were gradually able to recover after learning to meditate.

Meditation will help you relax, reduce or eliminate anxiety, and overcome any destructive behaviors you may be struggling with.

If you make meditation a part of your everyday life, you will feel better, more positive, relaxed, peaceful, and happier. You will improve the gray matter of your brain and feel more in control of your mental health.

Meditation and Physical Health

Over the past decade, a consensus has emerged from medical professionals: chronic stress causes numerous health-related problems, including high blood pressure, decreased immunity, and impaired cognitive functions. Fortunately, by reducing stress through meditation, you can improve your health in all of those categories.

Your cortisol levels matter. Cortisol is considered nature's built-in alarm system and is your body's main stress hormone. It works with certain parts of your brain to control your mood, motivation, and fear. Cortisol is best known for helping fuel your body's "fight or flight" instinct in a crisis, but it also plays an important role in several other things your body does.

After the pressure or danger has passed, your cortisol level should calm down. Your heart, blood pressure, and other body systems will get back to normal.

Enter meditation.

According to a 2013 study by the journal *Health Psychology*, the practice of meditation was shown to have an impact on the reduction of cortisol. The study followed its participants for three months, and their cortisol levels were measured before and after the study. The study found that after regular meditation, cortisol levels trended downward.

When you reduce your stress, you can then begin to realize the more specific effects of meditation on your health.

High Blood Pressure

Hypertension, or high blood pressure, can be a deadly condition that leads to heart attacks, strokes, and heart disease. Keeping your blood pressure in check is critical for maintaining good health on these fronts.

Meditation helps you relax. And when you are relaxed, meditation helps reduce your blood pressure. In one study, when patients were taught to meditate to relax, more than 60 percent lowered their blood pressure as a result.

Dr. Randy Zusman at Massachusetts General Hospital agreed. He explained on National Public Radio that prescribing meditation for patients with high blood pressure could lead to a reduction in the need for blood pressure medication.

Your Immune System

Your immune system is a complex group of processes in your body that fight infection and disease. A vigorous immune system is crucial to living a healthy life.

Stress and anxiety wreak havoc with your immune system, making it more likely that you will become sick.

Recent studies have shown that meditation can also play an integral role in maintaining and even strengthening your immune system. For example, according to researchers at the Infanta Cristina Hospital in Spain, meditation was shown to increase the level of white blood cells that fight off viruses and bacteria.

New studies are coming out on a regular basis that show the positive impact meditation has on the immune system. A study conducted by the Harvard Medical School showed that individuals who practice meditation have better immune systems. Another study done at UCLA found that meditation in older adults could prevent the expression of a group of genes that activate inflammation, improving the immune system from another direction.

In other words, meditation can make you less sick.

Meditation, Chronic Illness, and Pain

Chronic pain can be debilitating. To relieve it, doctors commonly prescribe opioids, which are pain-reducing chemicals that can have devastating side effects and are highly addictive.

A 2016 study found that a meditation practice can significantly reduce the intensity and the unpleasantness of pain in the body.

The journal *Neuroscience* reported that you can save money on prescription drug costs while simultaneously relieving pain more effectively. Meditation works. I have seen it in my own life. After a double discectomy (back surgery), I eliminated all pain medication within forty-eight hours.

I take more than a few drugs for multiple sclerosis, and I can tell you personally that medications can have bothersome and debilitating side effects. This isn't true with meditation. There is no pain, addiction, or side effects. None.

Jon Kabat-Zinn, the creator of the Mindfulness-Based Stress Reduction program, agrees that medications play an important role in medicine. But he also warns against the casual, habitual, or mindless use of any chemicals (be they prescribed, legal, or illegal).

Kabat-Zinn's research shows that meditation could be a useful tool for managing chronic pain. Meditation has become a medical treatment.

Always check with your medical provider before making changes, but a regular meditation practice may be able to help you reduce the amount of medicine you have to take for chronic pain and live a better-quality life.

Meditation, Relationships, and Quality of Life

Millions of people practice meditation. It is no longer seen as a "hippie" practice that involves sitting in silence. And with new studies coming out every year, the benefits of meditation seem to be endless.

Meditation helps you become more resilient, and resilience allows you to live a happier, higher-quality life. Meditation can be incredibly therapeutic.

A study from the Finnish Institute for Health and Welfare calculated the effects of multiple risk factors, including lifestyle-related ones, on the life expectancy of men and women. Heavy stress shortens life expectancy by 2.8 years, according to ScienceDaily.

Meditation and Crisis

Every now and then, your life can be turned upside down because of a crisis. And crises need to be dealt with. I have had my fair share of crises in my life, and I am sure that plenty more will come. Almost nothing can prepare you for what will unfold in your life when a crisis happens. The timing is always bad.

Stress, anxiety, and ongoing racing thoughts have become a common part of our lives. Many of those thoughts stir up physical sensations and experiences that result in stress, tension, or anxiety.

Kirt Baab, a psychotherapist and meditation and yoga instructor with the Cowell Family Cancer Center, says that our minds go through three stages during a crisis.

When you are in crisis, your thoughts and feelings are like cars traveling along a busy freeway. They are always going to be there because that is the nature of the mind. The only difference is that sometimes the freeway of the mind is busier than at other times. It is when we get caught up in the traffic of the mind that our stress and anxiety levels rise.

While crises are rarely something we wish upon ourselves, the opportunity they bring is what we learn as a result of how we handle them.

The popularity of meditation is increasing as more people discover its benefits.

The benefits of meditation include better focus and concentration, improved self-awareness and self-esteem, lower levels of stress and anxiety, and fostering kindness. Meditation also benefits your physical health, as it can improve your tolerance for pain and help fight substance addiction.

Meditation is something everyone can do to improve their mental and emotional health, so why not you? Let's get started.

How to Get the Most from Your Meditation Practice

What is a beginner's mind?

According to Wikipedia, a beginner's mind is described as having an attitude of openness, eagerness, and lack of preconceptions when studying a subject, even at an advanced level, just as a beginner in that subject would.

A beginner's mind involves dropping expectations and preconceived ideas about something and seeing things with an open mind. If you've ever learned something new, you can remember what a beginner's mind is like. You might have been confused because you didn't know how to do whatever you were learning, but you were also looking at everything as if it was brand new, perhaps with curiosity and wonder. That is a beginner's mind.

The beginner's mind is an attitude of getting started, experimenting, and learning along the way.

To get the most from your practice, adopt a beginner's mind. Here are some ways that you can develop a beginner's mind:

- Take one step at a time.
- Fall seven times, get up eight times.
- Do not prejudge.
- Live without *should*.
- Keep an open mind about how to apply what you learn.
- Find an appropriate time to implement each new thing you learn.
- Let go of the desire to be an expert.
- Experience each moment fully.
- Discard the fear of failure.

With a beginner's mind, you will be more open to what is new to you.

Consistently Meditating

As a kid, did you ever hear someone say, "Practice makes perfect"? Have you ever played a sport, either alone or with others? You practiced over and over. Meditation is the same.

It is estimated that approximately 15 percent of people in the United States have tried meditation. The keyword is "tried." But most have not stuck with it.

Meditating one time won't help much with stress. Realizing results requires consistency, patience, and a commitment to the practice of meditation. We know this, but people still give up.

But why?

People new to meditation often worry that they are doing it wrong. The newness of meditation overwhelms them. However, meditation is not about getting it perfectly right. It is about taking a seat, getting started, learning, and meditating every day.

Patience is a habit, and when we are not patient, we get frustrated. Frustration is the emotional energy that causes us to quit. When we are impatient while learning to meditate, we can't come to our seat with the right attitude.

Consistency develops routines and builds momentum. It forms habits that become almost second nature.

Great meditation practices are developed by doing the work and not giving up when a session isn't perfect. When you feel a lack of progress, take a seat again. You don't need to know everything. You just need to know what to do next. Take baby steps.

Successful meditators set themselves up for success by having a beginner's mind. They take the next step, over and over, until it is second nature.

Remember how I asked you to create a goal in the

beginning? Coming back to your intention and your desire to decrease your stress will help you stay consistent.

I suggest that you grab a piece of paper or a calendar and write out a simple plan to meditate.

Going to meditate daily? Then write it down. Are you going to meditate for a set period of five or ten minutes? Write it down. Your plan doesn't have to be long or filled with lots of detail. A written plan of your intentions will keep you on track.

Meditation is to your mind what yoga and exercise are to your body. Whether you feel it or not, your meditation practice will support you all day long. Practice it daily because the greatest results come through patience and consistency.

When Should You Meditate?

My proprietary method of meditation is called Easy to Meditate for a reason. Anyone can do it at any time, in just minutes per day.

There are no rules that say you must meditate at a specific time of day or night. Pick a time that works for you. Don't pick a time when you feel hurried or under duress.

When you wake up, your brain is still quiet, so why not prime the pump first? Early morning peace and quiet have positive effects. Nearly everyone is still asleep. There are no distractions. Like an early morning cup of coffee, meditation can bring you clarity and ease.

I recommend that you meditate in the morning. When you enter your day having meditated, you feel good. It is amazing what this feeling can do for your outlook on the day.

However, you can meditate during the day, night, or any time when you feel the need to calm down, reset, or get balanced. The key is to be consistent.

How Long and How Often Should You Meditate?

To receive the benefits of meditation, you must have a regular practice. Meditating for a few minutes a day is better than not meditating at all. Meditating for a longer period is more beneficial than a shorter one. The most important thing is to meditate regularly.

I often hear a particular question and get variations of it all the time: "How long do I need to meditate for?"

If you are just starting out, I recommend that you meditate for just a few minutes every day. You can start with as little as one or two minutes.

When you can sit still for that long, then move to five minutes and then to ten minutes. Keep increasing your time as you get comfortable with the practice. The most important thing is to just start. You are trying to set a new habit, so start small and simple and build consistency.

Decide on a length of time you will commit to every day. If possible, start meditating every morning for just a few minutes and, if you can, every evening for a few minutes. A meditation practice is like brushing your teeth.

Because everyone is different, there is no one right amount of time to meditate each day when you are established. The more time you invest in your practice, however, the more results you are going to see.

Meditating for just five to ten minutes a day has been shown to have a positive impact. Meditating for twenty minutes or longer has been shown to have even more benefits, so this would be a good goal to aim for if you can.

Practice meditation every day. When a daily meditation practice isn't achievable, you can still enjoy some benefits from meditating three to five times a week. Meditating daily, however, will help you create a habit and get you the most results.

Where to Meditate

The key to creating consistency is to find a place you're comfortable with—a place that resonates with you and that you can make your meditation spot.

Consider turning one of your rooms into your meditation room. A spare bedroom or loft area could be a great place to meditate, as could a corner of your bedroom or living room. Choose a place that isn't too noisy. Whether it is a spare room, a closet (make sure that it is big enough), or a corner of a room, pick a space you can come back to over and over. Ensure that you are comfortable.

A single space that you use again and again is preferable because you can customize or adapt it. It will become familiar. You are anchoring your habit in your space and setting yourself up for long-term success.

A meditation space can be as simple as setting out a cushion in a room of your home where you always feel peaceful. The whole point of meditation is to remove stress from your life, so don't create extra stress by trying to perfect your meditation space. It can always be moved or adjusted based on your needs or desires as you go.

The Meditation Practice

Here is the step-by-step Easy to Meditate approach:

1. Choose a nice, quiet, and comfortable place where you won't be disturbed for three to twenty minutes or longer. A place where you are comfortable will make the practice easier.
2. Dress comfortably—nothing tight, nothing restrictive.
3. Sit down, relax, and rest your hands on your lap. Sit in a comfortable place with your back straight. Sit quietly, and either close your eyes or focus on an object in front of you. Take a minute or two to settle yourself.
   → You can sit on the floor with the support of a meditation cushion or on any chair with your

feet resting on the ground. It isn't necessary to force yourself into any uncomfortable position.
    → Regardless of how you sit, maintaining the natural curve of your back is important. That means no slouching. If you have chronic back problems and cannot sit for a prolonged period, try another position or use a pillow.
    → Adjust your position if necessary.
4. Exhale and relax your muscles. You shouldn't experience discomfort during meditation. The goal is to be comfortable and focused.
5. Take a few slow, gentle, deep breaths, inhaling through your nose and exhaling from your mouth. Don't force your breathing. Let it come naturally.
    → Your first few breaths of air are likely to be shallow, but as you allow more air to fill your lungs each time, your breaths will gradually become deeper and fuller.
6. Focus your attention on your breathing. Continue to focus on your breath for as long as you like.
    → If you find your attention straying away from your breaths, gently bring it back. Your attention may wander many times.
7. Just stick with it. This can sometimes be easier

said than done. Getting your mind to cooperate can be like house-training a new puppy.
   → It isn't easy, but it can be done. Don't give up. Stick with it.
8. When you are ready to end your meditation session, open your eyes and stretch.
9. Don't jump up immediately. Take a moment to appreciate that you took the time to slow down and take care of yourself.

Remember to enjoy your practice. Every meditation is not going to be perfect. Starting your practice may not seem easy at times, but it is worth it. Keep an open mind. Take the time to appreciate that you are doing something good for yourself and practicing self-care.

Creating a Habit

Developing any new habit can be difficult. However, if you are serious about improving yourself through meditation, you must make it a part of your daily routine. The benefits and rewards that you will gain by developing a daily meditation practice will compound as time goes on.

If you miss a day, that is okay. Not preferred, but okay. Just start again the next day.

In 2010, a study conducted at University College London showed that it takes an average of sixty-six days to build a new habit. This means that you need to consistently meditate for about two months.

I suggest that you set aside a regular time every day to meditate. To help you build the habit, set a reminder or a trigger that reminds you to perform your meditation practice every day. I have found that the easiest way to do this is to incorporate meditation into your morning routine before your day gets busy. However, you can meditate at any time that makes sense for you.

You may experience times when you don't want to continue meditating or you feel it isn't paying off. This happens. Stay with your practice anyway.

Track your progress and stay accountable. There is an old saying: "Whatever gets rewarded gets repeated." To help get your meditation habit to stick, reward yourself. It can be as simple as giving yourself a pat on the back or a drink like a cup of coffee or an iced tea.

Try using a meditation log, like a smartphone app or a paper log. Keep it simple and easy to use. It must be convenient.

Consider using an accountability partner or hiring a coach. When someone holds you accountable, you will find it more difficult to skip a meditation session. People who have accountability are often far more successful than those who don't.

Whenever possible, enjoy your practice. It isn't a job; it is a part of your lifestyle and a way of taking care of yourself. Meditation is a habit that is worth starting and sticking with. It will give you clarity and focus, and it will bring calmness into your life.

Meditation can be a momentum builder for the rest of your life if you make it a habit.

The Monkey Mind

Sometimes in meditation, you may feel blank or empty, like nothing is happening. This is good. That sense of calm and stillness is something you should strive for.

However, sooner or later, you will run into something called the "monkey mind." The term "monkey mind" refers to a restless, chaotic, confused, and unsettled state of mind. Different people experience it in different ways.

However, everyone who meditates goes through periods where they start feeling an inner crazy energy. It is normal. Our minds tend to jump from one thought to another. We feel like we are going in a hundred directions.

Numerous scientific studies have revealed that we experience between 50,000 and 70,000 individual thoughts every day. Many of our thoughts are irrational fears, which contribute to our stress. Although you may have gotten used to the racing thoughts and see them as normal, they contribute to your stress. Monkey mind will not hurt you, and it will not ruin your day, but it will make it harder. Taking space away from it in meditation is part of what gives you calm.

Don't be surprised by the sudden urges that you will get during your practice. Some of these urges include:

- Getting up
- Putting on the television or radio
- Eating
- And more

Resist these urges and keep meditating.

These and other urges happen to everyone at one time or another, to both new and more experienced meditators. Resisting them is part of the practice of meditating.

When You Hit a Wall

After practicing meditation for a while, many feel they hit the proverbial wall. Hitting a wall feels like coming up against an obstacle that stops your progress. It feels like losing momentum. We have all been there, feeling stuck and thinking we just can't go on.

However, everyone hits a wall in meditation (and our lives) now and again. It is normal. Personally, I felt this after meditating for approximately six months.

In this section, I'm going to help you get over the hump. Here a few ways to take your practice to the next level when you feel like giving up:

1. Meditate for a longer or shorter period. With Easy

to Meditate, I teach people to start their meditation practice or habit with just a few minutes. If a few minutes is no longer working, why not increase the time to ten, fifteen, or twenty minutes or longer? There are no fixed rules to how long you can meditate at a time or the number of times a day you do. Change things up.
2. Focus on the quality of your meditation habit, not the quantity. Maybe you can change the place where you meditate. Try to change your breathing pattern.
3. You might want to include some soft background music.
4. Meditate outside instead of inside.
5. Meditate with a group instead of alone. The experience of meditating in a group is quite different than practicing on your own and is a great source of inspiration and support.

Sometimes you will just need a bit of variety. Indulge yourself. Develop a habit that you enjoy, not despise.

Getting Support

You might be one of the lucky few who have a supportive family and group of friends who will drop everything when you feel stress, rush over to be with you, and let you curl up into a ball next to them while they hold your hand. But most of us do not.

Just reading this short book will put you miles ahead of most people who try to develop a meditation habit without the right guidance. But most of us will need more support.

So where do you go for that support? Join a community. You can practice meditation on your own without the support of others, but there is something very powerful in being part of a community of people who are going through the same journey you are.

At Meditation Not Medicine, we have formed a supportive community where you will find inspiration for your daily practice. You also have the option to sign up for the Easy to Meditate coaching program. This program is designed to hold your hand and walk alongside you. It will help you create a successful meditation practice that will help you deal with your stress without the woo-woo, empowering you to manage your stress in new ways.

There you will find a digital course and a website with lots of tools and a supportive community. You can learn from the comfort of your own home or from another favorite place in an easy way.

Visit www.meditationnotmedicine.com and join the community today.

Almost Done

After decades both in the corporate world and as a business owner, I have seen a lot. At times, the level of stress I both felt and witnessed was overwhelming.

I spent time and money trying to eliminate my own stress and witnessed others do the same. The consequences were not always positive. My multiple sclerosis diagnosis drove me to find an answer.

I read books, did deep web research, and talked to medical professionals, trying to find a solution—and I eventually did. After years of meditating, I am a different person. I have learned so many valuable lessons. I wish someone had made meditation easier for me in those early days. Easy to Meditate was created with you in mind. The system is not only easy, but it can also be tailored to you and your lifestyle. I wanted to share what I have learned.

Stress is an epidemic in our society. It is causing us needless suffering. It causes anxiety, depression, physical health problems, chronic illness, and pain. It strains relationships and your quality of life.

Let me review what we covered earlier in this book:

- The Epidemic of Stress
- Stress, Mental Health, and Physical Health
- Stress, Chronic Illness, and Pain

People, both young and old, who meditate daily experience less stress and anxiety and live happier and healthier lives.

However, to help reduce stress, you must address it head-on. You must respond and not react. You must practice meditation daily and consistently.

In the meditation section of this book, we covered the following:

1. What Is Meditation?

2. Meditation, Anxiety, and Depression
3. Meditation and Physical Health (including high blood pressure and your immune system)
4. Meditation, Chronic Illness, and Pain
5. Meditation, Relationships, and Quality of Life

If you are serious about improving yourself through meditation, you must make it a part of your daily routine. The benefits and rewards you will gain by developing a daily meditation practice will compound as time goes on.

Fortunately, learning how to meditate and developing a daily meditation practice doesn't have to be difficult. In fact, it is Easy to Meditate.

I am grateful for you. Thank you for joining me on this journey.

Acknowledgments

First, I'd like to thank God, who created this life just for me and who has given me a gift in the form of a lesson. I am deeply grateful and ask that you help me change the world one person at a time.

I cannot express enough gratitude to my wife, Haley, and my two sons, Andrew and Daniel. They have never looked at any of my challenges—medical, physical, or other—as a burden or challenge to them or to our family. They have never seen me as sick or disabled, but instead as a person who can overcome any obstacle.

Haley, Andrew, and Daniel, you are my light and my heart. You are my greatest teachers, and I am grateful to get to share my life with you. I dedicate this book to you. I love you. Thank you for inspiring me to be the best person I can be and for allowing me to be the best example that I can be for you.

To my sister, Ruthi, for always being by my side and having my back.

Thank you to all my family, both immediate and extended, and to all the friends who have stood by me all these years. You are few but true.

Thank you to everyone who assisted in providing material for this book—a group that is unfortunately too numerous to mention by name. I am indebted to the many experts whose teachings and shared knowledge have been included in these pages.

And lastly, thank you to the readers and students who have believed in me and granted me their trust. I am honored to be part of your journey.

About the Author

ADAM WEBER is the "NO BS, common sense" speaker, author, product creation specialist, and owner of the highly successful companies Weber Real Estate Advisors and Weber Advisory Group.

Adam is a former corporate warrior with a progressive form of multiple sclerosis. He helps others learn to deal with their stress through his proprietary form of meditation, called Easy to Meditate, in person and online.

He is a New York native now living north of Manhattan with his wife, Haley, and his two sons, Andrew and Daniel. When he's not in his home office, you can find him with his Golden Retriever–English Setter mix, Churchill.

To learn more about Adam and Easy to Meditate, visit www.meditationnotmedicine.com.

www.ingramcontent.com/pod-product-compliance
Lightning Source LLC
Chambersburg PA
CBHW030529080526
44586CB00011B/368